How to Start
a *Successful*
Medical Billing
Business

By Alice Scott &
Michele Redmond

The materials contained in this book are provided for general information purposes only and do not constitute legal or other professional advice on any subject matter. Solutions Medical Billing Inc does not accept any responsibility for any loss which may arise from reliance on information contained in this book. We have given the most up-to-date information available.

The authors disclaim any personal liability, loss or risk incurred as a result of using our advice, information, or methods, either directly or indirectly.

This publication provides our opinion in regards to starting a medical billing business. We in no way intend to render legal, accounting or any other professional advice.

Regarding licensing a business enterprise or any other legal, accounting, contractual or tax matter, we strongly suggest that you seek, when necessary, the services of an appropriate licensed professional and comply with licensing requirements in your community.

The authors disclaim any personal liability, loss or risk incurred as a result of using our advice, information, or methods, either directly or indirectly.

Revised September 2009
Revised September 2007
Revised February 2006

Copyright 1999
by Solutions Medical Billing Inc.
8251 New Floyd Rd
Rome, NY 13440
(315)-865-4299
(315)865-6359 fax

Other books available by Alice Scott and Michele Redmond – available at our website www.medicalbillinglive.com

"Basics of Medical Billing" - Instantly Improve the efficiency and cash flow of your office using this guide! It's a must read for everyone from the receptionist to the doctor in any medical office!

"12 Marketing Strategies to Grow Your Medical Billing Business" – written in 2002 and revised in 2007. If you've started your medical billing service and need to find more clients, you **need** this book.

"Take Your Medical Billing Business To The Next Level" – Are you ready to expand your medical billing business? Are you ready to take on more business or hire an employee? Here are the secrets we've learned in the last 14 years from starting our own medical billing business to currently billing for over fifty providers.

"How to Complete a UB04 Form Completely and Correctly" – Complete instructions on completing a UB04 form correctly so your claims will be paid on the first submission.

"How To Complete a CMS 1500 Completely and Correctly - Line By Line, Box By Box". – Complete instructions on completing a CMS 1500 form correctly in easy to understand language.

"Mental Health Billing Made Easy" – How to make sure your claims are paid properly and you are reimbursed completely for your mental health services. Whether you are a social worker, a psychologist, a psychiatrist or a psychoanalyst, this book can teach you exactly how to bill out and get paid for your services

"Chiropractic Billing Made Easy" – How to make sure your claims are paid properly and you are reimbursed completely for your chiropractic services. This book can teach you exactly how to bill out and get paid for your services

Table of Contents

Introduction

What is a medical billing service?

The purpose of this book is to help you to avoid some of the mistakes we made in starting our electronic medical billing service in 1994. Prior to starting our business, Michele had worked for five years for an insurance company processing medical claims, and I had run my own business for over 25 years.

We thought it would be no problem, but boy did we have a lot to learn. We purchased an expensive package which was supposed to teach us everything we needed to know to make a fortune at medical billing, but unfortunately the program was a total loss.

This did not stop us. We persisted, we have learned much, and finally made our business a success, but, we learned the hard way mostly by trial and error. You too can be a success at medical billing by learning from our experiences.

You will need to learn what equipment you need to start your service, how to choose software, how to find clients, what to charge, what to say and do on your first appointment, what your work actually consists of, what you need to know about codes, and how to actually get started.

This book is designed to give you all the information you will need to get off to a great start. It will **not** teach you how to do medical billing, but it **will** teach you to start a *successful* medical billing business. Best of luck in your new venture!!

Our Story

Michele and I started our medical billing service in 1994. When I first saw an ad for medical billing at home, I gave it to my daughter, Michele, who had been working for an insurance company for the last 5 years at a very stressful job. She called the number and received an informational packet about a medical billing package that cost around $5000.

She was ready to start a family and wanted to work at home, but she had never run her own business. That's where I came in. I had run my own business for over 25 years and was now looking for a new opportunity. I didn't know anything about insurance billing, but we figured as a team, we would be great.

We sent away for several other packets on similar packages and we started comparing the offers and found they ranged in price from $4000 to $10,000 and in training from two days to five days.

Some companies offered their own clearing houses which seemed like a savings. Most offered the necessary software. We spent a lot of time comparing companies, checking with the Better Business Bureau, and doing research to see what would be our best option.

We chose a company in Atlanta that charged $5000 and booked our flights for the two day training. We were excited. However, after the two day training, we didn't know much more about this business than before we went.

The package was useless. The software was produced by the company itself; therefore it was not compatible with any clearing house other than their own, which wasn't sending any claims electronically at that time. They were sending the claims on paper.

We didn't get any useful information from them as far as starting our business, getting accounts or doing follow up. Most of the time was spent training us on their software.

Now we were $10,000 in debt and still at square one. We started over. After logging on to a bulletin board service strictly for medical billing, we received a lot of information on different software and clearing houses. We sent for demos and purchased Lytec Medical and Dental.

We got some marketing tips and made a few friends. We did anything and everything we could think of to get some clients. When we say anything and everything, we mean it. We were very creative in our initial marketing.

Our first account was a new doctor who knew less about insurance billing than we did, which turned out to be a blessing. We didn't make much money, but we were getting experience and that's what we needed.

Medical billing was much different at that time than it is today. The internet was new and did not have a lot of information available on the subject. Packages such as the one we purchased were very common and mostly scams that preyed on people like us to just wanted to start their own business.

We made some mistakes in the beginning because we had nowhere to find information. We learned a lot by trial and error, and we had a few laughs along the way.

Now people call us all the time asking for our advice on getting started in their own medical billing business.

We decided the best way to share the information was to put it all together in a manual – exactly "how to" start and run a *successful* medical billing business. We wrote this manual so you can refer to it often when your next question comes up.

It contains what you will actually need to get started and build a successful business. With our success we found a desire to help others get off to a great start.

We have revised this book quite a few times to keep up with the changes in the industry. What worked a few years ago is antiquated now and there is a need to put new systems into place.

Technology has changed a lot in the last few years offering the medical biller many new ways to save time and money. This business is constantly changing and with the change is the necessity to keep up and stay competitive. It is important that the beginner know what he or she is getting into and what to expect in this business.

Getting Started

What do I need to get started?

The key to any successful business is research. In order to establish a successful business, you must build a good foundation.

Without a good solid foundation, your business will crumble to the ground with the first challenge it faces. In order to build a good foundation, you must research the field of medical billing thoroughly.

It is crucial that you completely understand the business if you are going to succeed.

There are several places you can go to begin your research. One of the best places to get information on medical billing services is from other people who have already done it.

This book is a great place to start! It is one of the main reasons we wrote it. When we started, we tried to talk to other local services. We didn't look at it as being competitive. Unfortunately they did!

We have met other billing service owners at a local insurance seminar who were located about 1 ½ hours away from us and they were open to sharing information. If you can find a way to connect with someone in person, whether local or a little ways away, it could be very helpful to you.

Another place to find other medical billers who will share information is on the internet. Watch the medical billing forums for great questions and answers to the problems we are dealing with every day. Our forum is located at www.medicalbillinglive.com/members . We get some great threads going on marketing, starting your business, and getting your first clients. Our readers are not afraid to share their experiences and knowledge.

You can access websites for software and actually download demos to find one that you are comfortable with. You can shop for office furniture and supplies. You can read about current medical billing topics in ezines like http://www.ezinearticles.com. You can research medical billing courses and even take courses online. Here is more information on a course we recommend www.solutions-medical-billing.com/medicalbillingcourse.html.

You will have to invest some money to get your medical billing business started. There is some equipment you will require. Medical billing software better known as a practice management system can cost thousands of dollars. You'll need a fax machine and a dedicated fax line. You will need a photocopier, desk, chair, good lighting, phones, answerphone, file cabinets and more. Make sure you look into all options as some of the newer technology can save you lots of money.

But this business can give you the freedom you may be looking for. The most difficult part of this business for most beginners is signing up those first clients. It's not the work involved or learning the new software. It's getting the clients. If you are determined to make this business work for you, nothing will stop you.

Today there are many places to find help with questions in the medical billing field. There are many courses available, books to read, and websites to gather information. Choices are better than ever in software and equipment.

See what it takes to get your business up and running. Besides our free forum, we offer a subscription to our free newsletter offering information on current topics at http://www.solutions-medical-billing.com. We will help you get started. You can also find more of our ebooks available at www.medicalbillinglive.com.

Internet

The internet can be a very useful tool in starting your medical billing business. As stated in the previous section, you can get a lot of research done on the internet. In doing that research, you may make some contacts that you will want to stay in touch with as you establish your business.

As web based software has developed and improved, it has become possible for this new technology to save incredible amounts of time and money. Server based practice management systems like Lytec and Medisoft have become antiques. Web based programs offer amazing options never before available. Unfortunately web based programs can be very expensive so make sure you check out the options before you commit.

Most insurance companies have websites that you as the provider's representative will need to access. Some of these websites offer a convenient place to check benefits on patients, verify ID#s, check claims status, submit adjustment forms, and much more. Many companies have their newsletters and/or bulletins available on-line. The newsletters contain valuable information regarding billing and you will want to make sure you read these.

Many forms are available on these websites that you will find useful. If you have a provider who wants to become participating with the insurance company or needs to update or change information, the forms are usually available on-line.

Some electronic transmissions require the internet. For example we submit our N Y Medicaid claims via the internet. We create our file of Medicaid claims and upload it directly to Medicaid via their website. Of course, you would need a high speed connection in order to use it for this purpose.

We also use the internet to look up NPI numbers, phone numbers of an insurance company or a doctor if we do not have it on file. We've also found it very handy when we need to send flowers or a gift to a provider.

As you can see, the internet is an important tool in starting your medical billing business. Also important is having a high speed connection. Of course having the internet connection opens up your medical billing data to viruses and hackers. Make sure you have good virus protection, pop-up blockers, firewalls, spam blockers, etc. to insure proper security for your information.

Computer and Printer

Computers are developing at remarkable speeds. Your computer is your livelihood. If you are buying a new one, shop around. Talk to the salesmen. Tell them the requirements of your medical billing software. Computers get outdated very quickly, so don't buy the one that just meets your requirements.

All the experts also suggest you do not use this computer to download games. This computer is for your business needs.

Be prepared to upgrade your computer system at least every four years. Make sure it has a good backup system as it is very important to keep your information backed up daily.

Make sure you consider all that you will need in a computer. Besides size of the hard drive and memory you will need a high speed connection and a modem.

You will want a decent monitor, probably at least 17". Remember, you will probably be spending a lot of time looking at that screen.

The printer is also very important as you will be doing a lot of printing. You may have thought you wouldn't need a printer as everything goes electronic, but that is not reality. Many secondary claims must be printed. Most no fault and workers comp claims must be printed. EOBs must be photocopied and submitted with secondary and tertiary claims.

Make sure your printer meets all of your printing needs and is economical to operate. It can be difficult to calculate the cost of printing as many printers don't tell you, but the information is available on the internet and is important. You will find yourself making many photocopies and want them to be made at a reasonable cost.

Know what type of forms you will be printing. A laser printer is a little more expensive to buy, but saves you a lot in cartridges.

When we first started, we had to print 3 part Workers Comp forms so we had to use a dot matrix printer. Fortunately these forms are no longer required so we switched to a much more efficient laser printer.

This printer had two drawers plus a feed tray. It was very convenient as we keep HCFA or CMS forms in one drawer and plain paper in another. But then that printer became outdated. We now lease a large 4 drawer printer/scanner/copier. This machine does things we never thought of and at a cost of only 1.4 cents per copy plus the monthly lease fee.

We also offer credentialing services to providers. This is where we found some great advantages to the new printer we lease. We could now scan a credentialing packet after it was completed and email or fax it to a provider right from the printer.

Now we have the ability to scan any document and email or fax it wherever we please. This opened up a huge amount of possibilities to us. It is amazing the uses we find for this machine. The ability to scan documents allows us to scan claims and eobs and store them on the computer rather than in file cabinets.

If you need to print your own business cards or brochures to get started, you may need a color printer. Many of us who love photography have digital cameras with a color printer for the photos. You can use this printer to make business cards and brochures. Carefully think about what you will be printing when making your decisions.

Software

There are many good software programs available for medical billing. You want to make sure you get one that is capable of handling several doctors' offices and a variety of specialties.

The big difference between practice management systems today is whether they are server based or web based. Server based software is installed on your computer while web based software is accessed on the internet. Web based software also is available as ASP or SAAS.

We used NDC Lytec Medical for many years.. They are reasonably priced and easy to use and kept up with our needs until web based software became available at a reasonable cost. We now find that a web based program can save us much time and money as it is so much more efficient.

Your software package can cost you from $1000 to tens of thousands of dollars. Demo's can be downloaded from the Internet. Make sure you choose a software program that you are comfortable using. Also available are some specialty software programs for chiropractic, mental health, physical therapy, etc.

In software terms, do you need a single user or milti-user software? You don't want to buy a single-user software if you plan for your business to grow and have more than one user. Or at least make sure you can upgrade to the multi-user version without too much hassle or cost.

There are many things you will want to take into consideration when choosing your software. Do you plan on doing all the billing yourself or do you want to grow into a larger billing service with multiple employees? You do not want to have to change software in the future and try to get all your information transferred from one program to another.

Web based software is available with price based upon how much volume you expect to do. Your agreement with the software vendor will probably lock you into a certain time frame. You can expect to commit to a year's service.

Some web based software is priced per seat or by how many computers will be accessing it at the same time.
As of this writing (September 2009) we are using Xena-Health web based software in Beta version and are excited about how much time and money it will save us over our old server based Lytec system. You can call us for more information on Xena.

Does your software come with CPT and ICD9 codes available to import? This isn't a big deal if you are billing for small specialty providers, but if you have a larger medical practice – this can be huge. Entering all the ICD9 (diagnosis) codes and CPT (procedure) codes can be tedious.

Software is not something you purchase and that's it. If you are in business for any amount of time (hopefully you aren't doing this for a six month time filler!!) you will need to update your software. The world of medical billing is constantly changing especially since HIPAA. Your software must be able to change with it. That's one of the great things about web based software. It can be changed on an ongoing basis not just when a new version is released.

Another important reason to pick a good solid company to purchase your software from is for support. You may find yourself in a position where you can't get your software to do something you need it to, or you are having a problem with your software. You will need to be able to contact the company for support and the support needs to be good.

When you purchase your software, find out if you are purchasing it directly from the company or from a reseller. Usually the price is the same, but the reseller may offer support that the company doesn't.

If you purchase a medical billing package that comes with software, you will need to see if that software is compatible to any clearing house or if you will be locked into using their clearing house which may not fit your needs. See our chapter on Clearing Houses. Choose your software and clearing houses carefully. They are big decisions to make.

Once you have your software installed in your computer, or have accessed your web based program, practice with it. Learn to get around in your program. Enter some fictitious claims. See how the program works. Read the manual from cover to cover. Familiarize yourself completely with the program. You need to get comfortable with using the software.

In our original search for a web based software, we found most were cost prohibitive for our needs. We were billing for about 60 providers at that time and many companies charged a monthly fee per doctor that was more than we charged some of our smaller providers. We would have had to give up all our small accounts in order to make it work. On top of that most of these companies charged a hefty up front fee ranging from $5000 to $22,000. It was out of the question.

When SaaS technology (Software as a Service) evolved, web based software changed. We found a company that charged no up front fees or per provider fees. This company developed their software for the medical billing service market. They charge only a monthly fee based on the number of computers accessing the program. Here is more information on this software www.solutions-medical-billing.com/medicalclaimsbillingsoftware.html

Phones and phone lines

You will find you require at least two phone lines – one land line for your telephone and another for your computer and fax machine. High speed internet is a must for your internet needs but some of our claims go through the modem and telephone line.

We find that a land line rather than a cell phone is necessary for your business needs. Cell calls can be very staticky, noisy and unreliable. When you get a potential client on the phone you want to be sure to have a clear connection.

Keep your personal line separate from your business line. You do not want to have your business line tied up with personal calls. Do not allow children to answer your business phone unless you have trained them to do it in a professional manner and they are capable of taking a message and getting it fully in tact to you.

Check the various services available with your phone company. We had rollover on our first line which means that if we are talking on line one, another incoming call will automatically rollover to the second line if it is not in use.

You will find that physician's offices do not like to call and get a busy signal so you want to make sure you have at least two lines available. We eventually found it necessary to add a third and fourth and fifth phone line which we then used for the computer modems and outgoing calls so our other lines were not tied up.

Some people like to use call waiting instead of the expense of the extra line and rollover. We find this is not very professional. Sometimes it is impossible to interrupt a conversation in time to get the other call if you're the only one in the office. The other caller then doesn't get an answer or even an answer machine or worse yet, a fax noise in their ear.

If you have a second line with rollover, the first person can actually hear the other phone ringing. It sounds much better if you say "Please hold so I can get the other line."

Get yourself at least one good two (or more) line phone. There are many options available and phones are relatively inexpensive now. We also find that a headset is invaluable for getting work done while you are on hold with an insurance company. A speakerphone option is also a must for us.

As you grow, you may want to consider a phone system. The initial cost is a little high, but if you grow to have several employees and you're not all sitting in one big room, a phone system is great. It allows you to intercom between phones, transfer calls, and have individual voice mails.

Before we switched over, we would have to yell to each other when a phone call came in! It was not very professional.

We were lucky with our first phone system. We bought it used from a provider we billed for who had shut down an office. If you find yourself ready for a phone system and cost is an issue, watch the classifieds for a used one or even check Ebay.

We are now in the process of changing our whole phone system once again. It is important to keep up with the changes in technology to find the best alternative to your needs. Our phone bill was getting very expensive so we started looking into the options.

Our local charges for the five phone lines was over $250 per month. Our long distance charges including our 1-800 line had grown to over $200 per month. We were spending almost $500 per month for our phones.

Our office manager looked into the options and decided on a voice over computer system where there were no long distance charges. All calls were included in the monthly fee along with voice mail for each phone. There was also no need for all the extra lines. Each phone will be accessible at the same time without the use of extra lines.

The exciting part about this new system besides the savings is that we won't have to answer the phone any more unless the call is directed to our individual extension. Sometimes our phones are ringing all day. These constant interruptions to the girls answering the calls and transferring them to the correct person were interfering with productivity.

Clearing houses

In order to submit claims electronically, you must choose a method to transmit the claims to the insurance companies that will work best for you. There are a couple of different options available.

One of these options is using the services of a clearing house. The second is using free software offered by the individual insurance carriers. The third is purchasing the software to file direct to the insurance carrier.

Clearing houses have changed a lot in the past few years. They now offer many more services with bigger benefits for the user. Costs vary greatly between different clearing houses, so calculate your estimates carefully when you make a decision.

Many times a practice management system will be tied to a particular clearing house. This doesn't necessarily mean that you must use that clearing house but it is important that you find out. They may strongly encourage you to use the clearing house they are linked to but you may be capable of submitting to other clearing houses if you choose.

When claims are sent through a clearing house they are routed electronically to the appropriate insurance company. Most clearing houses charge a fee. You are then limited to the insurance carriers that this particular clearing house accepts and any other claims must be printed to paper.

Most clearing houses post the list of payors or insurance companies that they submit to on their website. You should check over the list to make sure that the major carriers you will be billing to are on that list. If won't do you any good to sign up with a clearing house that doesn't submit to the carriers you need.

Many clearing houses offer services in addition to just electronic claims submission. Some offer online eligibility, electronic remittances, and claim status checking. It is important that you know all the services you will be signing up for and the fees you will be charged.

Sometimes the print to paper is an option offered for an additional cost by the clearing house. They are then printed and stuffed into envelopes and mailed to the insurance carrier.

Some insurance companies offer free software that will allow you to submit claims to them electronically. Usually the free software option means double entry of the data. It is usually a stand alone program and you have to enter all of the data in your practice management program for tracking purposes and in the stand alone program to submit the claims.

Other insurance carriers have an online claim submission option through their website. Usually you have to register or sign up and then you can submit claims directly through the website. This is also considered electronic submission but will require you to also enter the information in a practice management system for tracking purposes.

A third option is to purchase software which will allow you to act as your own clearing house. The software is usually a little pricey, sometimes costing as much as your practice management program, but when you are billing for a large number of providers, it is worth it. With this method the claims are batched by the separate program through your practice management system and then submitted directly to the insurance carriers.

Not all insurance companies have the capability to receive insurance claims electronically. These companies generally require that their claims be submitted on CMS 1500 forms.

The clearing house will do this for you for a charge, it's called turning them to paper, but it may be more efficient and cheaper if you print those on paper (HCFA 1500 form) and send them directly to the insurance company yourself. You need to compare the clearing house fee to your expenses. When you are printing and mailing yourself, you can fit many claims in one envelope if they are all going to the same address.

Most clearing houses charge you to submit claims electronically. There are some free ones out there but they usually have a limited list of insurance carriers they can submit to.

You must decide the most practical method of sending your claims electronically and be willing to change if a better method becomes available. One thing you will learn about this business is that things are always changing and it is important that you stay aware of the changes and keep up with technology.

In choosing a clearing house there are several things you will be looking for.

- ✓ Do they have a minimum requirement?

- ✓ Is there a set up fee?

- ✓ What is the cost per claim?

- ✓ What do they charge to turn a claim to paper?

- ✓ Do you get confirmation that the claims went?

- ✓ Do they submit to the carriers that your providers bill?

- ✓ Do they send you error reports?

- ✓ What type of scrubber do they have for up front editing to prevent claims from being denied?

- ✓ How will the clearing house bill you?

- ✓ If you have a problem and need to speak to someone, how do they answer phone calls or do you have to leave a message?

Code Books

You will need to keep current CPT code books. They are published yearly. Code books cost between $50 and $150. There are many suppliers of these code books. www.amazon.com is a good place to search. CPT codes are copyright protected by the AMA and cannot be copied.

ICD9 codes however are not copyright protected and can be found on various websites by doing a google search for current ICD9 codes. We are currently using http://www.icd9coding1.com/flashcode/userRegister.do and have found it to be quite reliable.

Codes are changing every year and it is necessary to keep on top of them. Depending on the specialties of the providers you work with will determine if you need to order new ones each year.
If you only work with say chiropractors, you may not need to purchase a CPT book every year.

HCPCS code books may also be required for some providers. HCPCS are another form of CPT codes used for certain services such as drug administration, immunizations, entral therapy, and durable medical equipment.

There will be many changes in coding in the next few years including moving to ICD10 codes. The current ICD9 codes are too limited for modern day reporting and we are the only country still using ICD9s.

Certification is available in medical coding and may be required in the future in order to code claims correctly.

HCFA 1500 UB04 and Workers Comp forms

Even if you are sending your claims electronically, you will find that you need HCFA 1500 forms. They are the standard insurance claim filing form used by most medical providers and insurance carriers. These are available in one, two or three part, carbonless pages and in tract feed or plain sheets from several different suppliers.

The forms you choose will be dependent upon your needs. We started with two part tract feed forms, but found it only made for a lot of unnecessary paper storage.

We now use only single page HCFA's. If we should need a copy for any reason, the information is in the computer and we can easily reprint one. Make sure you choose a HCFA form that will work with your printer.

HCFA's can vary greatly in price and are less expensive when purchased in quantity. If you want to compare costs, check some prices here http://www.solutions-medical-billing.com/cms1500.html.

Workers comp insurance claims must be filed differently. In NY they are not filed on HCFA 1500 forms but a special form called a C4 which is available from the Workers Comp Dept. Whenever a person is filing a workers comp insurance claim, this C4 form must be completed.

There are currently two separate C4 forms available. One is for the initial visit and reports how the accident occurred and what is involved. The second form is for subsequent visits.

Physical therapists and occupational therapists file workers' comp claims on a slightly different single page form called an OT/PT-4.

Once a workers comp claim form is completed we print two copies. We send one to the insurance company and the other goes to the workers comp office.

We do not keep copies of these forms since we can print another one easier than to find one in a file cabinet if we need to resubmit.

Some software actually creates the C4 form and you only need to print them on white paper. If your software does not print the form, you can usually download a form off the internet and print your own.

If you are unable to download the form or just chose not to, you can purchase the forms preprinted. Check with your State Workers Comp Board to find where to order these forms.

Desk, chair, typewriter, photocopier
fax machine and filing cabinet

You will need a good sized computer desk and comfortable chair. You will be spending a lot of time in this chair and want to avoid unnecessary trips to the chiropractor. The desk needs to be large so you can spread out your work.

You will also need at least one large filing cabinet and lots of file folders. You will then need to set up a filing system. You will eventually have several different filing needs and will require several file cabinets.

You will be filing claims on whatever form they were sent to your office from the providers office as well as eobs after they are entered. Later on you may refer occasionally to these files to find certain eobs to resubmit a secondary claim. You also will be filing receipts for the business, credit card statements, and other important documents.

Keep each providers information separate. We keep one folder for claim information, one file for eob's, and one file for the provider information.

Every month we rotate the claims and eob files so they are current and anything you need to find from the past can be located. We write the dates in large black numbers on the front of each file folder.

We store records for the previous year in file boxes labeled so you can find something if need be. Be sure to label folders and boxes so you can easily locate the information you need.

How much we use our typewriter was amazing. It seemed as if the computer would make a typewriter unnecessary, but it is not so. We use it to type envelopes and sometimes we need it to fill out forms. It is not absolutely necessary to have a typewriter, but it sometimes makes things easier and more professional looking.

We also found we needed a photocopier. You can purchase a small used one for a few hundred dollars or rent one. Make sure you compare cost per copy when looking at a photocopier.

Generally speaking, the less expensive the copier, the more expensive the copies. You will be making a lot of copies.

We made do with a small copier for many years. Last year we leased a large photocopier/scanner/printer. What a difference it made to us. We were amazed.

The first thing we realized with the new machine was the amount of copies we were actually making. Now that we are paying per copy, we were shocked at the number of copies we actually print. The price per copy was much more reasonable than we were paying before. The toners were included in the monthly cost so we no longer had to pay separately for toner cartridges.

We also realized quickly how much time we had been wasting trying to keep our old printers working correctly. They would jam often, misfeed and just generally not print as well as they did when they were new.

Copying a stack of eobs or papers became much easier with the feeder option on a larger machine. This was another big time saver. We now had the options of collation and even stapling.

Next we realized what the scanner option could do for us. We could now scan any document to an email or fax address and send it from the machine. It was amazing what this opened up for us.

We offer credentialing services to providers. With the capabilities this new copier/printer offered us, we could now become much more efficient with our credentialing services. We can scan completed applications to the providers saving the cost of mailing.

A fax machine is also a necessity. We receive much of our billing over the fax and communicate frequently with our providers by fax. Sometimes an insurance company will ask you to fax an unpaid insurance claim to them.

Our first fax machine lasted only four years. Our second fax machine was a laser and was much more economical to operate.

We can still use that fax machine for outgoing faxes, but we now receive our faxes directly into our office manager's computer. She then prints them out. We can also receive faxes directly to the printer/copier. We aren't using that option right now, but we do any 1-800 faxes through the printer/copier.

When we changed our phone system over to the voice over internet, all long distance calls are free so if we scan any long distance faxes and send them to our email, we can send the long distance faxes free of charge, too through the email.

Business cards and brochures

You will need some professional looking business cards and brochures. Business cards are relatively inexpensive. You may want to hire a printing and graphics business to do these or you can do them up yourself on your computer very inexpensively.

The benefit to doing them yourself is that you can change them as you need to. You may decide to do a brochure on dental insurance billing to leave at dental offices. A month later you may decide to target chiropractors. This way you are not paying a printer every time you want a small or large change in your brochure.

There are several good publishing programs available to make brochures, fliers, business cards, etc. Check them out in your software store. Microsoft Publisher is one.

There are also some very fancy papers available to dress up your brochure. You can find paper in office supply stores or order by mail from Paper Direct.

When we first started out, we used brochures for a lot of things. We sent them in mailings, we placed them in our local hospital's waiting room, and we handed them out when we made cold calls.

Answering machine or voice mail

There are times that you will be unable to answer the phone. It is very important that the caller is able to leave a message.

Whether you have an answering machine or voice mail, be sure to leave a clear message on your machine with the name of your company and an assurance that their call will be returned in a reasonable time frame.

Make sure your message sounds professional. If there is more than one of you working in the office, you may want to consider voice mail. Many answer machines have voice mail capability or most telephone companies offer the service.

Our new voice over internet system allows for confidential voice mail for each phone.

Mailing, Postage & Envelopes

You will find when you mail out your paper insurance claims that you often have several going to the same company. These can be mailed in one envelope as long as they are all going to the same address.

Some companies have several different locations. Make sure you mail to the proper location. Failure to do so can hold up payment on a claim.

When you get four or five claims in an envelope, it is necessary to know the correct amount of required postage. An electronic postage scale will come in very handy.

Otherwise, you find yourself going to the post office, waiting in line, and expecting the postal worker to weigh each envelope for you.

It is really an unnecessary expense to rent a postage meter machine. If you keep first class stamps on hand, you save yourself hundreds of dollars of expense per year in renting a postage meter when the scale is all you really need.

You can purchase one at any office supply store for under $100. We usually purchase about a month's worth of self adhesive stamps at a time. Be sure you get stamps to cover extra weight.

Our mail varies in weight from less than one ounce to over one pound. We purchase all the necessary stamps to cover these amounts.

In order to have all the necessary stamps, we purchase $.44 stamps, $.17 stamps, $.61 stamps, and $.78 stamps as well as $4.95 for flat rate envelopes for larger packages.

Postage rates and requirements changed drastically this year. The post office decided that it cost them more to mail larger and heavier envelopes than smaller ones so they started charging differently for different sizes of envelopes.

These changes required a major shakeup in our mailroom. (I should call it mail desk.)   Small envelopes are between 6 1/8" and 3 ½" in size. Once you go over this size, you are charged more than you would be for the same weight in a smaller envelope.

The second issue was the thickness of the envelope. Small envelopes could no longer be over ¼" thick. We used to put as many as 15 papers in an envelope. Now you can hardly fold 15 tight enough to keep the envelope less than ¼".

We ended up making a chart of two different sizes of envelopes and all the possible weights and exactly how many of each value of stamps to put on the envelope.

We use quite a few 6" x 9" and 9" x 12" envelopes when we have several claims that are being mailed at a time.

One big time saver we found was window envelopes designed for HCFA 1500's. You just fold the HCFA to fit the envelope with the insurance company address in the window. This saves printing labels.

Even though the majority of our claims are going electronically, we still mail hundreds of claims a week to insurance companies that do not yet accept electronic billing.

When we first started our business, we would pile all the paper claims in a bin. When we went to mail them, we found it took a long time to sort them and get them ready to mail.

The larger we grew, the worse the problem. We found that the best way to keep track of these is something I found at an office supply store. It is a cardboard box divided into 21 slots that are just the right size for 8 ½" x 11" claim forms.

We've labeled each slot and as we take the claims out of the printer, we file them into the proper slot. Twice a week we go through the claims, put them in their envelopes and send them off.

With the scale in our office to apply the proper postage, we can put the claims in our mail box and avoid a trip to the post office.

Office

One of your first decisions will be where you want to run your business. Will you work out of your home or rent an office?

Most people who start medical billing businesses do so in order to stay at home. If you chose to work at home, you will require an office or space where you can spread out.

If your children will be near when you are working, you will need space for them to be playing quietly while you are on the phone. Don't try to run your business off your kitchen table. With medical billing, it just won't work.

If you decide to rent an office, you will have extra expenses from the beginning. Some people feel that it looks more professional to have an outside office. Our feeling is that if you are doing a good job, the doctor doesn't care where you are working.

Wherever you decide to have your office you will need to consider how much space you will need. We have found that we needed several different work stations.

One section to actual work on the computer, another section for filing, a third section for typing, and a fourth section for doing the mail. You will find that even if you send the majority of your claims electronically, you will still have a lot of mail.

You will mail any non electronic claims, secondary claims, patient notes, patient bills, appeals, workers compensation claims, letters and no fault claims. Make sure you take all of this into consideration when choosing a location.

There are many tax advantages in owning your own business. You will need to check with your accountant to make sure you keep track of all the expenses that will be deductible on your income taxes.

Naming your business

The name of your business can be very important. Remember, you will be answering the phone many times a day with this name. Write down all of your choices and then say them out loud. This may seem childish, but it will help you pick a good name.

Your name should be relevant to what you are doing, yet it should set you apart from your competition. For example, if you were starting a vending machine business, you wouldn't want to name it Johnson Inc. No one can tell what kind of business it is

You also wouldn't want to call it Best Vending Machines because that doesn't set you apart from the competition. A name more like Sammy's Snacks would be good. It relates to what you do, but it's personable and different from the competition.

Check out the competition in your area and make sure you don't use an existing name. Check with your county clerk regarding registering your name.

Clients

The final requirement you will need to get your medical billing business started is clients. This can be the most difficult part of the process and one of the most important. There are many different ways to look for clients and we suggest you use several.

You first need to understand that you are asking a provider to trust you with their money. The payments from their insurance claims are very important to them and they do not easily give the job of collecting them to someone they do not know.

Usually the money does not actually come to you, it still goes directly to them, but you are now responsible for making sure that it is paid on time.

Many times it is difficult for a provider to let the billing go outside of the office because they feel they are loosing control. As you gain more experience, you will see the needs of the office and learn to help the provider overcome the fears they have of hiring a service.

Some providers will already be signed up with a service they but they are not happy. This provider may be looking for someone who can do a better job than what they are now getting. You'll want to look at what problems they are experiencing now and convince the doctor why this won't happen if you are doing the billing.

Some providers will be interested in hiring you because you are sending the claims electronically which will get their money to them quicker than if filed on paper.

It can be a costly and involved process to get a small office capable of electronic submissions. This provider may be looking for other options.

Keep in mind when looking for clients that some offices are so well run that they may not need your services. If one person has been responsible for the billing for a long period of time and has been doing it well, it is very unlikely they will think that you will do a better job.

It's a good idea to introduce yourself and let them know what you do, as eventually the situation in the office may change and they may be looking for an alternative. Also, you never know where a referral may come from.

Sometimes at first glance an office will appear to be running well, but upon a closer look you will find they have serious problems. In mot of these cases, they don't want to admit that they have any problems.

If you clearly see some issues, try to approach them from that angle but do it tactfully. They may be sensitive to the issue.

See our section on marketing to learn how to get clients.

Understanding Your Value to Providers

It is important to understand what it is that you do that makes you valuable to a provider's office. Until you really understand this, it is difficult to convince a provider that they should hire you. Providers can hire help to send claims directly from their own office. Why should they hire you?

Some will hire you simply because they want their claims to go electronically so they are getting paid quicker. They've found it complicated to do this from their office or maybe they don't even have a computer. In some cases, they've tried to do it electronically from the office and it didn't work out well.

You may get a provider to sign with you because he or she can't keep good knowledgeable help in their office. A new provider just out of school trying to open their own practice may hire you because he is keeping down costs of additional help at the beginning.

The longer you work in this profession, the better you will understand how valuable you can be to your providers. You will eventually consider yourself a consultant. As you gain experience in your field of billing, you will be able to offer suggestions to increase their income (and yours) and improve their efficiency.

An office may contact you because their receivables are way too low and they can't seem to figure out how to increase them. We once met with a Doctor who owned a family practice with three MDs and three NPs. They were a very busy office seeing 80-100 patients a day but they were barely bringing in enough money to keep the doors open.

The doctor himself wasn't even getting paid. Yet we had to convince him he needed us. Within six months of hiring us we increased his receivables 100%. As you can imagine, we are now invaluable to him.

Anyone can send claims to an insurance company, but it takes a professional to do medical billing. There is so much more to billing than just submitting the claims.

You must know the requirements of each insurance company, make sure all data on the claim is correct, including the coding and follow up on any unpaid or rejected claims. A billing professional knows how to get claims paid quickly and correctly and knows how to make sure a provider is getting paid the most for his services.

You are not just a billing service, you are a billing professional and also a consultant. You will not just submit claims for your providers, but you will maximize their receivables. You will make sure they get reimbursed for their services.

You must assure them that you do not loose claims to timely filing and that you follow through on all claims to get them paid. Remember, if you are charging a percentage, your income is directly dependent to how much money you collect for the provider.

There are many ways you can become invaluable to your providers in addition to doing a great job on their billing.

You can act as a consultant to them advising them of ways they can increase their receivables (and your). You can also help them with credentialing or recredentialing and address changes.

Many providers cringe at the sight of paperwork and they are very grateful to you for helping them out. Any of these little things you can do to help them out just helps to build a stronger loyalty which usually leads to a long term relationship.

One of our best accounts is an office with two doctors who had placed an ad in the local paper for a person with billing experience. We answered the ad and after talking to the doctor, he realized that if he hired us it would eliminate the need for a workspace for a new employee, a computer, and all the additional expenses of another employee.

We've been working with them for years now and they are thrilled and give great referrals for us. They don't hesitate to tell others how much money they save and how much we have increased their income.

Billing Knowledge

There are many places to get an education on medical insurance billing. This is indispensable in this business. One of the best options is to take a class in medical billing. If you decide to take a class, make sure it is taught by someone who has actually done medical billing.

There are some great online courses that offer a solid foundation for this business. You can learn more about one we recommend here www.solutions-medical-billing.com/medicalbillingcourse.html.

You need to have a good understanding of medical billing and be able to read an explanation of benefits to know if it was paid correctly and how to act on it if it is not paid correctly.

Many local colleges offer courses on medical billing and coding. Michele got most of her education by working for the insurance company and I got mine by listening to her. Whatever you choose, make sure you understand medical billing inside and out.

You can get some great experience working in a doctor's office doing his billing. Even if it is billing for a specialty, it will be extremely beneficial. Nothing beats actual experience.

Personally we don't feel that becoming certified at Medical Billing is necessary. In 15 years of business, we have not yet had a provider ask us if we were certified.

It certainly won't hurt you to become certified, but I wouldn't go to great extremes or expense to do so. Bottom line – providers want to know that you know what you're doing when it comes to his or her billing.

Introduction to Marketing

Marketing is the most important part of getting your business started. Without clients, you don't have a business. There are many ways to market your new business, but the most important thing is to keep an open mind to all possibilities. There is no one right way to market.

If you're new to this, it is a good idea to try many different techniques and find what you are comfortable with and what works for you. Whatever methods you use, it is best to be direct and honest.

We are always finding new ways to market. Referrals are by far the best, but when you don't have any clients yet, it is hard to find anyone to refer you.

The absolutely best way to market is by networking. You need to get out and meet people – people in the medical field. It is much easier to talk to someone about what you do at a social event than trying to get past a gatekeeper to talk to the boss.

Look through our chapter on marketing and keep your mind open. You may think of any idea we haven't tried yet.

Marketing

1. ***Start with the doctors you go to***. Ask your family practitioner how he is currently doing his billing? Is he satisfied with the time frame it takes to get payment? Does he have a good follow up system for payments? Is he filing electronically? Does he have any problem areas?

Does he have a lot of turnover of staff? Each time he looses his billing person, he has to find another and train her.

Check with each doctor you go to - your dentist, chiropractor, counselor, orthodontist, pediatrician, etc. Ask them if they know of any physicians who are having problems with their billing. Tell him you've started an electronic billing service and you are looking for clients. Ask if they have any suggestions.

2. ***Spread the word.*** Networking is absolutely the best way to find leads. Tell your friends, business associates, and acquaintances that you have started a new business and are looking for clients. Ask them if they know of any doctors offices that have problems with the billing. Ask them if they will speak to their doctors about you.

3. ***Join networking groups,*** business clubs, chamber of commerce, etc. You'll get to meet doctors, dentists, and therapists on a social level. They will be much more likely to be interested in what you do. Use the membership listings to find who is a potential client to target and then find a way to meet them.

4. ***Mass marketing*.** You can generate one letter in your computer and send it to all the physicians in your phone book. Make sure you send a well written letter and follow up a few days later with a phone call. Plan it so you leave enough time to do all the follow up within a few days.

5. ***Barter*.** You may be seeing a provider who is willing to give you part or all of his insurance billing in trade for services. Even if you are not receiving cash, it is important to actually get the experience of doing some billing when you are getting your business started.

7. ***Advertising.*** It's a good idea to get your business name listed in the yellow pages. You may wish to purchase a little advertising space. You can also advertise your business in any local medical publications or the newspaper. And remember, your business is not limited to geographical location. You can submit insurance claims for a doctor in California even if you live in New York. You may want to try advertising on the Internet.

8. ***Phone calls***. Some medical specialties such as social workers, chiropractors, etc. do not require employees. You can call their offices and leave an intriguing message on the answer phone telling them briefly about your service.

9. ***Help wanted ads.*** Follow the help wanted ads in the local newspaper. Watch for listings that are looking for medical billers. Be prepared to send a brochure and business cards. We even wrote up a resume for our company.

10. ***New Practices***. Watch for new doctors starting their practice. They are the most likely to need help. Many new doctors are ill equipped to handle all the business obligations along with the patients and are glad to find help. You may have to do a little extra for them besides their insurance claims, but in the long run, it should be worth it. Check the newspapers for ads.

11. ***Referrals.*** Ask for referrals. Once you are working with a doctor and he is happy with your service, ask if he would be willing to refer you to any of his associates. As your business grows, you will find that your new business comes from referrals. Make sure you thank and reward the person who sent you the referral. They are very valuable to you. We also offer incentives for referrals.

Some of the girls who work in providers offices know others from different offices that might be interested. We've given gift certificates to a good local restaurant to people for giving referrals where we signed up the account.

12. ***Brochures.*** You may want to try walking into some of the potential doctors offices with your brochures and see if you can talk to someone in charge. Be professional. Don't expect that you will be able to speak to the doctor, but if they are having a problem with their billing, they just might be willing to listen.

13. ***Website.*** In this day and age a website is almost a requirement. But if you are wise, you can use your website for not only as a marketing tool, but to earn you money. Be sure to visit our website at www.solutions-medical-billing.com. for ideas.

When you first start your marketing endeavor, choose a medical field and target that one field. Specializing in one field makes good sense for many reasons. You can become an expert in that specialty. This makes you valuable to other doctors in that field.

You have a limited amount of codes to learn. You only need to know the codes in that field, not the whole ICD9 and CPT books.

Eye doctors hang out with eye doctors, chiropractors hang out with chiropractors. The provider you are working for is more likely to refer you to another provider in the same field.

Aggressively market this field. Don't sit and wait for a doctor to call you back because you left a message on his machine. Keep marketing. Find ways to meet professionals in your chosen field socially. You're much more likely to get their attention.

If you are not getting enough business from that field, pick one more and work that field also. But if you take on one chiropractor, one social worker, and one family doctor, you are going to have a lot more to learn.

What do you charge?

There are several ways you can charge your clients. You can charge a monthly fee. When you don't have any experience yet, this can be difficult, because you will have no idea of how much work an account will be.

The second way is a per claim fee. Many times, when sending the insurance claims is the only service you are providing, this can be the best way to charge. You may get anywhere from $3.00 to $8.00 per claim for an average provider.

When you charge per claim, make sure you are clear on whether or not follow-up is expected.

Most offices will hire you because they also want the follow up taken care of as well as submitting the claims. It has been our experience that a percentage works best in most cases when we are also following up but unfortunately percentages are considered "fee splitting" and are against the law in several states.

Percentages will vary greatly. You should try to get an idea what providers in your area are paying. 7% to 15% seems to be the range. When we charge a percentage, the percentage is based upon what the provider actually collects as a result of our billing.

You may also want to consider a minimum monthly charge. We have a few accounts that are so small that they are not worth working with. Either they don't get a lot of insurance billing or they give us only one kind of insurance billing. A minimum fee helps this situation.

In some states charging a percentage is considered fee splitting and is illegal. Check with your attorney if you run into this problem. It is difficult to set a monthly fee on work you have never done so give some major thought to how you are going to price your services..

We used to charge a percentage of what was collected, but found that we had to change our methods. New York is a fee splitting state and you can get your doctors in trouble charging that way. We now offer a flat monthly fee or a per claim fee based on the amount of claims they expect to send us.

In our contract with our providers, we state that we bill on the first of the month and payment to us is expected within 14 days. It is rare, but you may find that you have problems collecting from some of your providers. You have already provided your services and deserve to be paid on time. You must act firmly with your clients about your pay. The longer you wait to take care of this problem, the worse it will get. We suggest a past due notice sent on the 15th of the month reminding them that payment is expected by the 14th.

Insurances

There are two general categories of health insurance, public and private. Public health insurances consists of Medicare, Medicaid, Champus (government insurance), and various others.

Private health insurance consists primarily of commercial companies, including, Blue Cross Blue Shield plans, and Health Maintenance Organizations (HMO's).

In many of both public and private insurances, a provider can be either participating or non-participating. This means that he can choose to accept a companies guidelines and fees for services or not.

If he chooses to, he becomes a participating provider with that company. Some benefits of participating are: payment is sent directly to the provider (instead of the patient), being listed in the company directory, claims receive priority in processing over non-participating providers, higher fee schedules in some cases, and lower out of pocket expenses for patients with that insurance.

Some disadvantages of participating are: accepting the fee schedule and treatment being dictated. The disadvantage of not participating is patients may receive little or no reimbursement for services and may choose to go elsewhere.

Each carrier differs dramatically in their fee schedules, and in their requirements for participation, treatment authorization, and claims filing.

Providers may choose to participate with some and not with others and may look to you for advice in making this decision. It helps to know the requirements and fee schedules of common insurance carriers.

Many carriers have a timely filing deadline. That means that you have a designated amount of time from the date of service in which you have to file the claim. The deadline varies greatly from company to company.

Some have a deadline from as little as 30 days from the date of service and others can go up to 2 years. It is important to know the filing deadline for each carrier.

The patient can authorize payment to go directly to the provider by signing an assignment of benefits statement. If the provider participates with an insurance carrier, in most cases, the payment will automatically go to him, whether the patient signs a statement or not.

But some companies will only send the money to the provider if they have a signed statement on file. This statement can be as simple as a line on the bottom of the patient information form that states "I authorize payment for services to be sent directly to <fill in provider's name>." This assignment of benefits is indicated in box 13 on the HCFA 1500 form.

It also important to have the patient sign a statement indicating that the provider has permission to release any medical information to the insurance carrier that is necessary to receive payment for the services provided.

For instance, if the insurance carrier requests medical records in order to determine if a service is going to be covered, the provider needs the patient's permission to send the records to the insurance carrier.

Again, this can just be a simple line along with the assignment of benefits statement that is something like "I authorize the release of any information to the insurance carrier regarding my treatment."

Many patients are required by the insurance carrier to pay a portion of their bill in the form of either a co-payment or co-insurance. If the patient has an HMO, they will have a designated co-payment that they are required to pay.

Some insurance plans require that the patient meet a deductible each year. This deductible must be satisfied by the patient before the insurance company will begin making payments on their claims. The patient is responsible for this amount and deductibles vary from plan to plan.

It is a good idea for you to familiarize yourself with the major insurance companies for your area. Most commercial insurance companies have provider representatives. Find out who your area provider rep is and make contact with them to introduce yourself.

Medicare, Medicaid and many commercial carriers publish monthly bulletins or newsletters for the providers containing updates and changes. It is important to keep up with this information.

You can call the Medicare & Medicaid offices to see if you can get on the mailing list for these bulletins or ask one of your providers to save them for you when they are finished. Many of the bulletins or newsletters are available online.

It is a possible that a patient may be eligible for two separate insurance plans. One would be primary and should be billed first and the other would be secondary. Insurance companies determine which policy is primary through a method called COB, or coordination of benefits.

There are a couple of different methods to determine which insurance policy is primary. If a husband and a wife both work and both have family insurance policies, their own insurance will be primary and their spouse's insurance will be secondary.

When children are involved, one method used to determine who is primary is called the birthday rule. That is where the insurance plan of whichever person's month of birth is earlier would be primary. (If they are born in the same month they go on to the day of birth.)

Another method, called the gender rule, states that the male person's insurance plan is primary. Yet another would be if a person had two insurance plans themselves, one from a company that they are currently working for, and one that they are retired from, the insurance plan for the current employer would be primary.

If a person had an insurance plan and also Medicaid, Medicaid is always secondary to the other plan, no matter what it is.

When a patient has Medicare, Medicare is prime unless the patient or the patient's spouse is currently employed and has insurance coverage through that employer. The patient's coverage through the company of the employed person would be primary and Medicare would be secondary.

There is one exception to this rule. That is if the employed group insures less than 100 people, then Medicare would be prime even though either the patient, or the patient's spouse is employed. Medicare would have to contact the other insurance carrier to get the information straight.

There are some other methods of determining COB, but these are the most commonly used.

After receiving the EOB from the primary company, you print out another HCFA for the secondary company, attach the primary company's EOB and mail it.

Medicare has a program called Medigap which automatically forwards claims information electronically to secondary carriers able to receive claims. If Medicare forwards the claim automatically, it will indicate that it was forwarded and to what insurance carrier right on the Medicare Explanation of Benefits Statement.

A few companies can now receive even secondary claims electronically. You must check with each company to see how to file the secondary claims.

Claims – Paper Vs. Electronic

There are many advantages to sending insurance claims electronically instead of on paper. Electronic claims processing (ECP) saves time, labor, money and paper. Many insurance carriers including Medicare are now requiring electronic submissions and don't allow paper claims without a special waiver.

There is no need to print up a HCFA, just type the information into your computer. The claim can actually be received by the insurance company within 24 hours.

Many providers are not yet using ECP but would be interested in the benefits. ECP cuts down on much overhead for insurance companies and a few companies are trying to mandate ECP and are offering many incentives.

Providers are looking into ways to send their claims electronically. In order to send claims electronically from their offices, they must have a fairly up-to-date computer, high speed modem, appropriate software, clearing house connection and an employee who knows how to operate all this. You can show them that your service saves them the work of updating their office and having an employee who is capable of electronic billing.

A paper claim must go through many steps before it reaches the person who is responsible for paying the claim. The claim is first sorted and routed, microfilmed and batched. They are then keyed into a computer, examined by an auditor, and accepted or rejected.

Electronic claims can be processed much quicker and with fewer steps. Payment is much quicker when claims are submitted electronically.

The state of Minnesota recently mandated electronic submission of medical insurance claims. If all goes well in Minnesota you can be sure that other states will quickly follow.

Interviewing with a provider

Wow! You finally have an appointment with a provider. Remember, a provider is not always a doctor. Many providers that need medical billing done are not MD's. There are social workers, physical therapists, optometrists, etc.

One thing to remember when meeting with a provider is that they are a person just like you. Do not be intimidated by their title. They may be very good at what they do, and may have gone to school longer than you, but they need someone who knows about billing to take care of their receivables, and that someone is you.

What to wear: Dress business like. First impressions are very important. This meeting is most likely what the provider will use to make his decision as to whether or not to hire you. You want to be neat and professional. You want your appearance to show him that you run a tight ship. Arrive a few minutes early, but not too early. Your time is valuable too.

What to take: We like to be totally prepared when we go on an interview. We usually take a contract with us filled out with the providers name and address and a form for all the information that is required to begin working for a provider.

There is quite a bit of information that you will need and you want to remember as much as possible. Our intention is to sign him up and we like to be prepared.

Also in our folder we will have any paperwork we would need to file to get started. This may include a form to get permission to send the providers Medicare electronically and any forms from private insurances or the clearing house might require. A few business cards and a brochure will round it out. If you have any letters of referral from some of your existing clients, you may wish to bring copies of them.

Be confident: You provide a very good service, one that the provider needs. If he is already doing his billing in the office, you need to show him that you can do it more effectively and efficiently.

You are going to cut down on processing time, rejections, and claims that are "lost in the mail". You are also going to be able to follow up on claims faster because this is your only job. You don't have any patients to take care of, just the provider's billing. The more confident you look, the better your chances of getting hired.

This position is too important to not have someone who knows what they are doing - a professional. If it is a new provider, you can convince him that he is getting someone with experience. This will save him from having to hire someone and train them to do something that he knows nothing or little about. You can help him to get his practice going quicker.

Try to let the provider do most of the talking. Listen to what his needs are. Ask questions. Is he having any problems in particular? How would your service most benefit him?

It is easier to sell yourself when you know what his needs are. For example, if he has a high turnover rate, then you can emphasize that you are a reliable service that he can count on to be around. He won't have to bother interviewing any more people, and training them and hoping that they know what they are doing. Convince him that his receivables are too important to take a chance on.

Confidentiality is a major issue with many providers, especially with the new HIPAA laws. Your provider needs to be assured that his patient's information will not go beyond you and his records are kept in a secure area.

You must be very careful to not talk to anyone about any of your clients or their patients. And if you have anyone helping you, you must get them to sign a confidentiality agreement.

If he decides to go ahead and sign your contract, complete the necessary paperwork, thank him for his decision, advise him on how long it will take to get the necessary paperwork to go through and determine when and how you will receive your first claims.

Contracts

One of the first questions most people have when they start a medical billing business is what do they use for a contract. Many people ask us for a copy of our contract so they can get an idea of what they want to say. We used to use a very simple one page contract that really didn't say much. As we got more experience, we saw more things that we wanted included in our contract.

You must remember that your contract is protecting you. When you are first starting out, you may not be sure of what you want to be protected from. As you grow, you see more things that should be covered in your contract.

One of the most important things your contract will cover is how you will be paid for your services. Many billing services charge a percentage of the money collected. Before you charge a percentage, make sure your state does not have "fee splitting" laws which prohibit a provider from sharing any percentage of his income with anyone outside of a partner. The states we are aware of that have fee splitting laws are NY, Fl, and NC.

Other methods of charging are a per claim fee, a flat fee, or a certain dollar per hour amount. However you have made arrangements to get paid it should be clearly spelled out in your contract.

Your contract does not have to be a 20 page fine print legal document. It just has to state the important points regarding the relationship between you and the provider.

If you are taking over the billing from another service, you will want to spell out the dates of service you will be responsible for. If a collection agency is used by the provider, your contract should specify if you will be reimbursed for any collections.

One of the most important items to cover in the contract is how your services will be terminated. You will want to specify a certain timeframe to allow for the change and to make sure you are paid for the work you did.

The information you have received from the provider is the property of the doctor and is often expected to be returned to the doctor. This should be written into the contract. You might want to specify a timeframe for this also.

We highly recommend you do not copy someone else's contract. You need to think your situation through and write down everything you can think of that could go wrong and cover it in your contract. Get your ideas together and take them to an attorney to write your contract.

Our information regarding contracts is not intended to be legal advice. Laws differ in each state and we urge you to check with your attorney when you write your contract. Please read our disclaimer at:
http://www.solutions-medical-billing.com/disclaimer.html.

Working with your first doctor

So, you have your first account. The provider has decided to use your service. There is quite a bit of information that needs to be exchanged between the provider's office and your office.

You can build a form to take with you to fill in with the provider's name, title, address, phone number, fax number, specialty, any other office locations, tax id number, NPI #, Medicare number, Medicaid number, Workers' Comp number, office hours, which insurance companies he participates with, who you will be working with and the best time to reach them. Any numbers issued by private insurance companies, referred to as legacy numbers are generally not required since the use of NPI numbers.

You will also need a list of the CPT codes the doctor bills out with the charges they bill. Some providers use superbills which will contain all the CPT codes. If the office is not using a superbill or is a new provider without a system in place, you may be able to design a simple superbill for the office.

Establish a good relationship with the person you will work with in the office whether it is the provider, the spouse, receptionist, nurse, or office manager. Compliment them whenever possible. Tell the provider what a great job this person is doing – if they are.

This person could make you or break you. Occasionally you'll find it very difficult to work with someone. Try to stick it through for awhile. Sometimes you can iron out the problems. Many times these employees don't last long.

Most likely you will have some insurance company contracts that the provider will have to sign. You will also need to sign your contract with the provider. Also, Medicare requires the doctor's signature in order to bill electronically on his behalf. Our local Excellus BCBS requires the doctor to sign electronic contracts before claims can be submitted.

You will want to have all this paperwork completed as much as possible before asking the provider to sign. You don't want to be trying to figure out the forms in front of him. It will make it look like you don't know what you're doing.

We use little self adhesive stickers that say "sign here" that work great for this. Once this paperwork is complete you can get started on the billing!

Going to work
Starting a New Account

You have your contract signed, you have all the necessary numbers from the provider, and your paperwork has been sent to the clearing house. The first thing that you need to do is to find out when they want to start. Hopefully it will be immediately, but some may want to wait until the beginning of the month, or the quarter, or some other circumstance.

Assuming it is immediately, you will have billing to do now. You will need to set up your software for the new provider. You will need to consult your software manual for this information.

Start by adding a practice. You will need to enter all of the provider's information into the software so that it will print out on the claims. This includes name and address, phone and fax numbers, tax id number, and NPI numbers.

Once this is done you may want to add the appropriate ICD9 and CPT codes for this specialty or your software may have the codes preloaded or the capability to import the codes.

You will also need to set up paper filing system for the new account. You will need to develop a system. We set up a file for each provider with 3 folders in it. One for a copy of the contract and insurance forms, one for the patient's information forms and billing, and one for the eob's.

You may occasionally need to go back to these files to retrieve something. What I recommend is always putting new papers in the back of the folder. That way you can try to retrieve things by date.

You will need to develop a system for each provider on getting the necessary patient and claims information to your office. This can be done many ways, depending on the number of claims, location of offices, specialty, and provider's wishes.

Some providers expect billing to be done daily, some feel monthly is often enough. Most of our accounts are sent weekly with some of our larger accounts being bi-weekly.

We receive claims information by mail, fax, email, pick up and drop-off. Each office can have a different method. Some of our providers are out of state and usually send us information by mail or fax.

We physically pick up information from our local offices once or twice a week. This works for us now, but we may find it easier to work with a courier in the future. A few offices fax, mail or email us the information weekly.

The important thing to remember here is to make it easy for your provider and your office. If they fax weekly and you don't receive a fax this week, make sure to call to find out why. If you can't pick up on a scheduled day, call and let your provider know and make other arrangements.

We receive the information in many different forms. Some offices that are already using medical billing software find it easiest for them to just print HCFA forms from their computers (on plain white paper to save costs) and send them to us. Other providers use a super bill. We have designed some of these super bills for them.

To a beginner, if a provider sends us a completed CMS form, it sometimes sounds like the providers office has done all the work already. Nothing can be farther from the truth. Claims must be tracked and checked for proper payment. Just printing a CMS form and mailing it out is only a small part of what is required.

We enter the information from their forms into our computer and either send them electronically or print HCFA's to send on paper. If a provider is using a super bill, it is necessary to also submit a patient information form to us containing patient demographics and insurance information unless the superbill contains that information.

Super bills can range from very simple to very detailed depending on the providers specialty. Super bills must contain patient name, date of service, services provided (CPT4 codes), and diagnosis (ICD9 codes).

If the HCFA's are sent to us, it is not necessary to use a super bill as the HCFA contains all the pertinent information. Once a patient is entered into our computer, we do not require the patient information sheet again. If the provider sees the patient on an ongoing basis, he will need to send only the claim information after the first time.

It is important to submit the insurance claims within 24 – 48 hours from when you receive the information from your client. You want the provider to get paid as soon as possible.

Some providers will expect you to do their patient billing as well as insurance billing. This needs to be addressed when you and your client agree on your services. If they want you to do the patient billing, there are a few things you will need to consider. Your billing software should give you a few options of patient statements.

Decide with your provider how often you will be sending out these statements and exactly what information he or she wants printed on the statement. Determine how long to let an account go before it is necessary to send it to a collection agency. You may want to strike up a strategic alliance with a collection agency, as they sometimes have the opportunity to refer your services to a provider.

We use a three statement patient billing policy. The first bill goes out with a detail of the charges and an explanation of what their portion is. You can purchase stickers with a variety of explanations, or you can make them up yourself with an inexpensive label program. Or you can print them directly on your statements.

Here are some examples of our most commonly used notes or stickers:

"Your insurance has paid its portion of these charges. The balance is your responsibility."

"These charges have been applied to your deductible."

"Your insurance states your coverage has been terminated."

If there is no response to the first bill, we send out a second bill 30 days later. That bill we print in a balance forward format and apply a sticker that says "2ND notice. We have not heard from you regarding your past due account."

If there is no response to the second bill, we send out a third and final bill 30 days after the second. That statement is also in the balance forward format and has a big orange sticker that says "Final Notice If payment is not received within 10 days, your account will be forwarded to collections"

This three statement policy is what we recommend to our providers, but ultimately it is up to them how they want their patient billing handled. Make sure you discuss this with them prior to doing any patient billing.

Another little trick we learned with patient billing is that patients tend to pay quicker if you include a return envelope in with the statement.

Many providers and services don't do this because they feel the envelopes cost too much. For the few pennies it costs for an envelope, the improved cash flow is well worth the expense.

We have a few very small accounts that we do patient billing. It isn't worth ordering 1000 return envelopes with their name and address so we simply make labels for these providers and apply them to small envelopes and insert them in the statements.

We take the patients statement and fold it so that the address shows through a window envelope with our return address preprinted. We then place the statement and the return envelope in the window envelope and mail it out.

You should pick a certain day of the month and designate it as your patient billing day. Pick a day that is not a busy time. For example, if you do your billing to your providers on the first of the month, you probably don't have time to do your patient billing then.

If you do your pickups on Monday, that probably wouldn't be good either. Consider making it the third Thursday every month.

Having good systems in place when you first start out will help you to run smooth as you grow.

Follow Up

Many people think that medical billing services just submit insurance claims for providers. They do that, but there is so much more.

After the claims have been submitted, you will need to keep track to make sure they are paid on time. If a claim is not paid in 30 days (longer for workers' compensation) you need to call that insurance company to see why it has not been paid.

You must also check rejection reports from your electronic billing. When you submit claims electronically, you will receive reports stating whether the claims were received, rejected or accepted and on some claims specific rejection reasons.

We have chosen to purchase software that allows us to act as our own clearinghouse and submit some of our claims directly. Others go through a clearinghouse. The initial expense was very high, but for the number of providers that we are billing for and the quantity of claims we submit, the direct filing method was the best option.

We receive two reports for each file submitted. The first tells us if the entire batch was accepted or rejected. The second report has a specific action on each claim. On the rejected claims, the report states the reason the claim was rejected.

Most clearinghouses will give you a variety of reports. The first one usually would be an initial rejection report, which would tell you if any of the claims were lacking necessary information. For example, if a patient's date of birth, or the marital status were missing, the report would indicate exactly what was wrong.

Then you should also receive a report which comes from the actual insurance carriers. This report would show you which claims were received, which claims were accepted (meaning there were no errors), and which claims were rejected. The claims that were rejected will also give you the reason for rejection such as "insured ID # invalid" or "patient's date of birth not match file."

You would then have to correct the information and resubmit the claim. If it comes back rejected, it's as if the insurance carrier never received the claim.

Ours is slightly different since we are acting as our own clearinghouse. We don't receive an initial rejection report because our software checks the claims for any lacking information before we even submit the claims.

We then receive reports from BCBS after the claims are submitted which tells us if a claim rejected after it was sent on to the insurance company and gives us the reason why. This report usually comes about 48 hours after claims submission.

You will be responsible for reading the explanation of benefit statements (Eob's) and performing any necessary action. The EOB is the statement that accompanies payment or denial of payment from the insurance carrier. If it is processed correctly, you will just need to enter the information, however if it processed incorrectly, you will need to take further action.

Insurance companies do sometimes make mistakes in processing claims. If you find an error, you need to call them and straighten this out.

A claim may be denied due to a coding error. If you have used an outdated CPT code, or an incorrect ICD9 code, you must submit a corrected claim. You may be able to appeal the claim with a phone call.

Another common denial is due to a request for additional information. You will need to get this information and forward it on.

Sometimes a written appeal is necessary. If a claim has been denied for late submission, you will need to type up a brief explanation as to why the claim was not submitted on time and send it to the insurance carrier with the denial.

On occasion a claim is denied because the insurance has been canceled. In this case, you must notify the provider immediately or if you bill the patients, send the patient a statement advising them their insurance has denied their claim.

It is your job to effectively read the EOB and act upon it to get the proper payment of each insurance claim for your client.

You can make yourself invaluable to your providers by your follow-up procedures. Set good procedures for follow-up right from the start and stick to them. Many providers don't have anyone in the office that really understands an EOB.

If you are unfamiliar with them, you should try to look at a couple to practice. If you have health insurance, you probably receive EOB's for your own family, but may never have paid much attention to them.

Most insurance companies send statements to the insured even if the payment goes to the provider. Get a few out and study them. The more you read, the better you become.

It is amazing that so many of the provider's staff do not know how to read these when they are so important. When you are trying to sell yourself to a provider, this can be one of your strong points.

Reports

Your software should be capable of generating several different reports. You will need to consult your software manual to see what reports are available to you. Some of the common ones are:

Insurance aging report - This report should list any outstanding insurance claims. Good software will allow you to sort your information in any way you wish. You can choose the aging by 30, 60, or 90 days and include or exclude certain data.

Patient aging report - This report will list any outstanding patient billing with options for sorting and aging. You will run this report when you send your patient billing.

Day sheet - This report will list all activities done on an account for whatever specified time frame. We use this report to bill our providers for our services when charging a percentage. We print it out on the first of the month and use the totals at the bottom to show amounts collected that month.

There are several others that you may find quite helpful. Your providers may wish to receive some of these reports once or twice a month. This is an area you can use to make yourself invaluable to your provider. One thing we find in many offices is that even if they are using medical billing software they do not know how to generate reports.

There is so much information that can be provided by reports. You can do a monthly analysis or a yearly analysis to let a provider know if they are on track. Or if not, where are they off?

Many providers are into the numbers and if you can provide them with the numbers, that makes them happy and it makes you look good. Familiarize yourself with your software's report capabilities.

HIPAA

HIPAA is the acronym for the Health Insurance Portability and Accountability Act of 1996. The Health Insurance Portability and Accountability Act of 1996 (HIPAA) mandated regulations that govern privacy, security, and electronic transactions standards for health care information.

These regulations will require major changes in how health care organizations handle all facets of information management, including reimbursement, coding, security, and patient records.

HIPAA calls for:

1. Standardization of electronic patient health, administrative and financial data

2. Unique health identifiers for individuals, employers, health plans and health care providers

3. Security standards protecting the confidentiality and integrity of "individually identifiable health information," past, present or future.

As a billing service, HIPAA will not impact you as much as the providers themselves, but it is important that you are familiar with it.

You must make sure that your clearinghouse is HIPAA compliant. If you are sending your claims directly to Medicare through their software, you should check with them to see if you need to do anything to become HIPAA compliant.

If you are just setting your business up, these things are probably already taken care of, but you should ask anyway, just to make sure. Any records that you have need to be either in a locked filing cabinet, or unable to be accessed by any outsiders.

You and any employees will need to understand the importance of confidentiality. Also, you should be able to advise your providers if they are breaking any HIPAA rules.

The following are some good informational websites regarding HIPAA:

http://www.hipaa-iq.com
http://www.hcfa.gov/hipaa/hipaahm.htm
http://www.hipaadvisory.com/

NPI Numbers

NPI or National Provider Numbers were implemented on May 23, 2007. Each provider must have an NPI number to identify themselves. Previous to the NPI number system, each insurance company would identify a provider with an individual legacy number.

In an effort to simplify healthcare administration each healthcare provider must obtain a free NPI number from the NPI enumerator to identify him/herself. Without this NPI identification number printed on insurance claim forms claims will be denied.

The original deadline for this requirement of the NPI numbers on insurance claims was May 23, 2007 but was extended to May 23, 2008 as many companies were not ready by the original deadline.

Any provider who is paid by insurance carriers for medical insurance claims or refers patients to specialists for treatment must obtain an NPI number.

A tax id number is also required besides the NPI number on all insurance claims. One of the services we offer as a billing service is that we will obtain the NPI number for our providers.

Terminology

Authorizations – prior approval of payment by the insurance carrier to the provider for services to a patient

Clearing house – A company which will receive electronic insurance claims, sort and reroute them to the proper carriers

Co-insurance – Portion of the insurance bill remaining after the carrier has made payment on a claim that is the patient's responsibility

Coordination of Benefits – Method of determining which insurance carrier is primary for a patient when more than one insurance is involved

Co-pay – Amount that patient is required to pay for each visit or service performed by a provider

CPT Codes – Physicians' Current Procedural Terminology is a listing of descriptive terms and identifying codes for reporting medical services and procedures

Crossover – Automatic forwarding of claim information from Medicare to a patient's secondary insurance carrier

Electronic claims processing – The process of submitting insurance claims electronically

Explanation of benefits - Statement which accompanies payment or denial of payment from an insurance company ICD9 Codes - International classification of diseases codes for purposes of diagnosis

Insurance Carrier - Insurance Company

Medigap - Medicare program that automatically electronically transfers claims information to secondary carriers

Modifiers - A two digit extension to a CPT code that further explains procedure or service performed

No fault - Insurance claims resulting from an automobile accident

Referrals - Notification from a patient's primary care physician for permission to go to a specialist (This is not always an authorization or a guarantee of payment)

Treatment notes (Soap notes) - Patient's progress notes

Superbill - A form used in a provider's office to document the patient's visit

Workers Comp - Insurance claims resulting directly from a work related illness or injury

Abbreviations

Auth/Ref - Authorization or referral

BC/BS - Blue Cross Blue Shield

BTW – Back to work

CAP - Claims Assistant Professional

CHAMPUS - Civilian health and medical program of the uniformed services

CMS – Centers for Medicare and Medicaid Services

COB - Coordination of Benefits

CPT codes – procedural medical code

Ded - Deductible

DOB - Date of Birth

DOS - Date of Service

DTW - Deep tissue work

Dx - Diagnosis codes

ECP - Electronic claims processing

EOB - Explanation of benefits

EOMB - Explanation of Medicare Benefits

ER - Emergency room

HCFA – Health Care Financing Administration

HCPCS – HCFA common procedure coding system

HIPAA – Health Insurance Portability and Accountability Act of 1996

HMO – Health Maintenance Organization

H & P – History & Physical

Lt – Left

MH – Mental Health

NF – No Fault
Non-par – Non=participating provider
OTR – Outpatient treatment report
PAR – Participating provider
PCP – Primary care physician
PI – Personal injury
POS – Place of service
PPO – Preferred provider organization
Pt – Patient
PT – Physical therapist
RNC – Reasonable, Necessary & Customary
ROM – Range of motion
Rt – Right
RTW – Return to work
Rx – Prescription for treatment
SOAP –
SOF – Signature on file
TX – therapy
UPIN – Unique Physician Identification Number
WC – Workers Compensation
2X – 2 Times
2X/wk – 2 times per week

Made in the USA
Charleston, SC
05 July 2013